INDIAN COOKBOOK 2021

DELICIOUS AND HEALTHY INDIAN RECIPES

SECOND EDITION

GORDON PHILIPS

Table of Contents

Kele ki Bhaji

(Unripe Banana Curry)

Ingredients

6 unripe bananas, peeled and sliced into 2.5cm/1in thick pieces

Salt to taste

3 tbsp refined vegetable oil

1 large onion, finely sliced

2 garlic cloves, crushed

2-3 green chillies, slit lengthways

1cm/½in root ginger

1 tsp turmeric

½ tsp cumin seeds

½ fresh coconut, grated

Method

- Soak the bananas in cold water and salt for an hour. Drain and set aside.

- Heat the oil in a saucepan. Add the onion, garlic, green chillies and ginger. Fry them on a medium heat till the onion turns brown.

- Add the bananas and the turmeric, cumin and salt. Mix well. Cover with a lid and cook on a low heat for 5-6 minutes.

- Add the coconut, toss lightly and cook for 2-3 minutes. Serve hot.

Coconut Kathal

(Green Jackfruit with Coconut)

Serves 4

Ingredients

500g/1lb 2oz unripe jackfruit*, peeled and chopped

500ml/16fl oz water

Salt to taste

100ml/3½fl oz mustard oil

2 bay leaves

1 tsp cumin seeds

1 tsp ginger paste

250ml/8fl oz coconut milk

Sugar to taste

For the seasoning:

75g/2½oz ghee

1cm/½in cinnamon

4 green cardamom pods

1 tsp chilli powder

2 green chillies, slit lengthways

Method

- Mix the jackfruit pieces with the water and salt. Cook this mixture in a saucepan on a medium heat for 30 minutes. Drain and set aside.

- Heat the mustard oil in a saucepan. Add the bay leaves and cumin seeds. Let them splutter for 15 seconds.

- Add the jackfruit and the ginger paste, coconut milk and sugar. Cook for 3-4 minutes, stirring continuously. Set aside.

- Heat the ghee in a frying pan. Add the seasoning ingredients. Fry for 30 seconds.

- Pour this mixture over the jackfruit mixture. Serve hot.

Spicy Yam Slices

Serves 4

Ingredients

500g/1lb 2oz yam

1 medium-sized onion

1 tsp ginger paste

1 tsp garlic paste

1 tsp chilli powder

1 tsp ground coriander

4 cloves

1cm/½in cinnamon

4 green cardamom pods

½ tsp pepper

50g/1¾oz coriander leaves

50g/1¾oz mint leaves

Salt to taste

Refined vegetable oil for frying

Method

- Peel the yams and chop into 1cm/½in thick slices. Steam for 5 minutes. Set aside.

- Grind the rest of the ingredients, except the oil, to a smooth paste.

- Apply the paste to both the sides of the yam slices.

- Heat the oil a non-stick pan. Add the yam slices. Fry on both sides till crisp, adding a little oil along the edges. Serve hot.

Yam Masala

Serves 4

Ingredients

400g/14oz yam, peeled and diced

750ml/1¼ pints water

Salt to taste

3 tbsp refined vegetable oil

¼ mustard seeds

2 whole red chillies, roughly chopped

¼ tsp turmeric

¼ tsp ground cumin

1 tsp ground coriander

3 tbsp peanuts, coarsely pounded

Method

- Boil the yam with the water and salt in a saucepan for 30 minutes. Drain and set aside.

- Heat the oil in a saucepan. Add the mustard seeds and red chilli pieces. Let them splutter for 15 seconds.

- Add the remaining ingredients and the boiled yam. Mix well. Cook on a low heat for 7-8 minutes. Serve hot

Beetroot Masala

Serves 4

Ingredients

2 tbsp refined vegetable oil

3 small onions, finely chopped

½ tsp ginger paste

½ tsp garlic paste

3 green chillies, slit lengthways

3 beetroots, peeled and chopped

¼ tsp turmeric

1 tsp ground coriander

¼ tsp garam masala

Salt to taste

125g/4½oz tomato purée

1 tbsp coriander leaves, chopped

Method

- Heat the oil in a saucepan. Add the onions. Fry them on a medium heat till they turn translucent.

- Add the ginger paste, garlic paste and green chillies. Stir-fry on a low heat for 2-3 minutes.

- Add the beetroots, turmeric, ground coriander, garam masala, salt and tomato purée. Mix well. Cook for 7-8 minutes. Garnish with the coriander leaves. Serve hot.

Bean Sprouts Masala

Serves 4

Ingredients

2 tbsp refined vegetable oil

3 small onions, finely chopped

4 green chillies, finely chopped

1cm/½in root ginger, julienned

8 garlic cloves, crushed

¼ tsp turmeric

1 tsp ground coriander

2 tomatoes, finely chopped

200g/7oz sprouted mung beans, steamed

Salt to taste

1 tbsp coriander leaves, chopped

Method

- Heat the oil in a saucepan. Add the onions, green chillies, ginger and garlic. Fry the mixture on a medium heat till the onions turn brown.

- Add the remaining ingredients, except the coriander leaves. Mix well. Cook the mixture on a low heat for 8-10 minutes, stirring occasionally.

- Garnish with the coriander leaves. Serve hot.

Mirch Masala

(Spicy Green Pepper)

Serves 4

Ingredients

100g/3½oz spinach, finely chopped

10g/¼oz fenugreek leaves, finely chopped

25g/scant 1oz coriander leaves, finely chopped

3 green chillies, slit lengthways

60ml/2fl oz water

3½ tbsp refined vegetable oil

2 tbsp besan*

1 large potato, boiled and mashed

¼ tsp turmeric

2 tsp ground coriander

½ tsp chilli powder

Salt to taste

8 small green peppers, cored and deseeded

1 large onion, finely chopped

2 tomatoes, finely chopped

23

Method

- Mix the spinach, fenugreek, coriander leaves and chillies with the water. Steam the mixture for 15 minutes. Drain and grind this mixture to a paste.

- Heat half the oil in a saucepan. Add the besan, potato, turmeric, ground coriander, chilli powder, salt and the spinach paste. Mix well. Fry this mixture on a medium heat for 3-4 minutes. Remove from the heat.

- Stuff this mixture into the green peppers.

- Heat ½ tbsp of oil in a frying pan. Add the stuffed peppers. Fry them on a medium heat for 7-8 minutes, turning them occasionally. Set aside.

- Heat the remaining oil in a saucepan. Add the onion. Fry it on a medium heat till it turns brown. Add the tomatoes and the fried stuffed peppers. Mix well. Cover with a lid and cook on a low heat for 4-5 minutes. Serve hot.

Tomato Kadhi

(Tomato in Gram Flour Sauce)

Serves 4

Ingredients

2 tbsp besan*

120ml/4fl oz water

3 tbsp refined vegetable oil

½ tsp mustard seeds

½ tsp fenugreek seeds

½ tsp cumin seeds

2 green chillies slit lengthways

8 curry leaves

1 tsp chilli powder

2 tsp sugar

150g/5½oz mixed frozen vegetables

Salt to taste

8 tomatoes, blanched and puréed

2 tbsp coriander leaves, finely chopped

Method

- Mix the besan with the water to form a smooth paste. Set aside.

- Heat the oil in a saucepan. Add the mustard, fenugreek and cumin seeds, green chillies, curry leaves, chilli powder and sugar. Let them splutter for 30 seconds.

- Add the vegetables and salt. Fry the mixture on a medium heat for a minute.

- Add the tomato purée. Mix well. Cook the mixture on a low heat for 5 minutes.

- Add the besan paste. Cook for another 3-4 minutes.

- Garnish the kadhi with the coriander leaves. Serve hot.

Vegetable Kolhapuri

(Spicy Mixed Vegetable)

Serves 4

Ingredients

200g/7oz mixed frozen vegetables

125g/4½oz frozen peas

500ml/16fl oz water

2 red chillies

2.5cm/1in root ginger

8 garlic cloves

2 green chillies

50g/1¾oz coriander leaves, finely chopped

3 tbsp refined vegetable oil

3 small onions, finely chopped

3 tomatoes, finely chopped

¼ tsp turmeric

¼ tsp ground coriander

Salt to taste

Method

- Mix the vegetables and peas with the water. Cook the mixture in a saucepan on a medium heat for 10 minutes. Set aside.

- Grind together the red chillies, ginger, garlic, green chillies and coriander leaves to a fine paste.

- Heat the oil in a frying pan. Add the ground red chillies-ginger paste and the onions. Fry the mixture on a medium heat for 2 minutes.

- Add the tomatoes, turmeric, ground coriander and salt. Fry this mixture for 2-3 minutes, stirring occasionally.

- Add the cooked vegetables. Mix well. Cover with a lid and cook the mixture on a low heat for 5-6 minutes, stirring at regular intervals.

- Serve hot.

Undhiyu

(Gujarati Mixed Vegetable with Dumplings)

Ingredients

2 large potatoes, peeled

250g/9oz broad beans in their pods

1 unripe banana, peeled

20g/¾oz yam, peeled

2 small aubergines

60g/2oz fresh coconut, grated

8 garlic cloves

2 green chillies

2.5cm/1in root ginger

100g/3½oz coriander leaves, finely chopped

Salt to taste

60ml/2fl oz refined vegetable oil plus extra for deep frying

Pinch of asafoetida

½ tsp mustard seeds

250ml/8fl oz water

For the muthias:

60g/2oz besan*

25g/scant 1oz fresh fenugreek leaves, finely chopped

½ tsp ginger paste

2 green chillies, finely chopped

Method

- Dice the potatoes, beans, banana, yam and aubergines. Set aside.
- Grind together the coconut, garlic, green chillies, ginger and coriander leaves to a paste. Mix this paste with the diced vegetables and salt. Set aside.
- Mix all the muthia ingredients together. Knead the mixture to a firm dough. Divide the dough into walnut-sized balls.
- Heat the oil for deep frying in a frying pan. Add the muthias. Deep fry them on a medium heat till golden brown. Drain and set aside.
- Heat the remaining oil in a saucepan. Add the asafoetida and mustard seeds. Let them splutter for 15 seconds.
- Add the water, muthias and the vegetable mixture. Mix well. Cover with a lid and simmer for 20 minutes, stirring at regular intervals. Serve hot.

Banana Kofta Curry

Serves 4

Ingredients
For the koftas:

2 unripe bananas, boiled and peeled

2 large potatoes, boiled and peeled

3 green chillies, finely chopped

1 large onion, finely chopped

1 tbsp coriander leaves, finely chopped

1 tbsp besan*

½ tsp chilli powder

Salt to taste

Ghee for deep frying

For the curry:

75g/2½oz ghee

1 large onion, finely chopped

10 garlic cloves, crushed

1 tbsp ground coriander

1 tsp garam masala

2 tomatoes, finely chopped

3 curry leaves

Salt to taste

250ml/8fl oz water

½ tbsp coriander leaves, finely chopped

Method

- Mash the bananas and potatoes together.
- Mix with the remaining kofta ingredients, except the ghee. Knead this mixture to a firm dough. Divide the dough into walnut-sized balls to make the koftas.
- Heat the ghee for deep frying in a frying pan. Add the koftas. Fry them on a medium heat till they turn golden brown. Drain and set aside.
- For the curry, heat the ghee in a saucepan. Add the onion and garlic. Fry on a medium heat till the onion turns translucent. Add the ground coriander and garam masala. Fry for 2-3 minutes.
- Add the tomatoes, curry leaves, salt and water. Mix well. Simmer the mixture for 15 minutes, stirring occasionally.
- Add the fried koftas. Cover with a lid and continue to simmer for 2-3 minutes.
- Garnish with the coriander leaves. Serve hot.

Bitter Gourd with Onion

Serves 4

Ingredients

500g/1lb 2oz bitter gourds*

Salt to taste

750ml/1¼ pints water

4 tbsp refined vegetable oil

½ tsp cumin seeds

½ tsp mustard seeds

Pinch of asafoetida

½ tsp ginger paste

½ tsp garlic paste

2 large onions, finely chopped

½ tsp turmeric

1 tsp chilli powder

1 tsp ground cumin

1 tsp ground coriander

1 tsp sugar

Juice of 1 lemon

1 tbsp coriander leaves, finely chopped

Method

- Peel the bitter gourds and slice them into thin rings. Discard the seeds.

- Cook them with the salt and water in a saucepan on a medium heat for 5-7 minutes. Remove from the heat, drain and squeeze out the water, set aside.

- Heat the oil in a saucepan. Add the cumin and mustard seeds. Let them splutter for 15 seconds.

- Add the asafoetida, ginger paste and garlic paste. Fry the mixture on a medium heat for a minute.

- Add the onions. Fry them for 2-3 minutes.

- Add the turmeric, chilli powder, ground cumin and ground coriander. Mix well.

- Add the bitter gourd, sugar and lemon juice. Mix thoroughly. Cover with a lid and cook the mixture on a low heat for 6-7 minutes, stirring at regular intervals.

- Garnish with the coriander leaves. Serve hot.

Sukha Khatta Chana

(Dry Sour Chickpeas)

Serves 4

Ingredients

4 black peppercorns

2 cloves

2.5cm/1in cinnamon

½ tsp coriander seeds

½ tsp black cumin seeds

½ tsp cumin seeds

500g/1lb 2oz chickpeas, soaked overnight

Salt to taste

1 litre/1¾ pints water

1 tbsp dried pomegranate seeds

Salt to taste

1cm/½in root ginger, finely chopped

1 green chilli, chopped

2 tsp tamarind paste

2 tbsp ghee

1 small potato, diced

1 tomato, finely chopped

Method

- For the spice mixture, grind together the peppercorns, cloves, cinnamon, coriander, black cumin seeds and cumin seeds to a fine powder. Set aside.
- Mix the chickpeas with the salt and water. Cook this mixture in a saucepan on a medium heat for 45 minutes. Set aside.
- Dry roast the pomegranate seeds in a frying pan on a medium heat for 2-3 minutes. Remove from the heat and grind to a powder. Mix with the salt and dry roast the mixture again for 5 minutes. Transfer to a saucepan.
- Add the ginger, green chilli and tamarind paste. Cook this mixture on a medium heat for 4-5 minutes. Add the ground spice mixture. Mix thoroughly and set aside.
- Heat the ghee in another pan. Add the potatoes. Fry them on a medium heat till golden brown.
- Add the fried potatoes to the cooked chickpeas. Also add the tamarind-ground spice mixture.
- Mix thoroughly and cook on a low heat for 5-6 minutes.

Bharwan Karela

(Stuffed Bitter Gourd)

Serves 4

Ingredients

500g/1lb 2oz small bitter gourds*

Salt to taste

1 tsp turmeric

Refined vegetable oil for deep frying

For the stuffing:

5-6 green chillies

2.5cm/1in root ginger

12 garlic cloves

3 small onions

1 tbsp refined vegetable oil

4 large potatoes, boiled and mashed

½ tsp turmeric

½ tsp chilli powder

1 tsp ground cumin

1 tsp ground coriander

Pinch of asafoetida

Salt to taste

Method

- Peel the bitter gourds. Slit them lengthways carefully, keeping the bases intact. Remove the seeds and the pulp and discard them. Rub the salt and turmeric on the outer shells. Set them aside for 4-5 hours.

- For the stuffing, grind together the chillies, ginger, garlic and onions to a paste. Set aside.

- Heat 1 tbsp oil in a frying pan. Add the onion-ginger-garlic paste. Fry it on a medium heat for 2-3 minutes.

- Add the remaining stuffing ingredients. Mix well. Fry the mixture on a medium heat for 3-4 minutes.

- Remove from the heat and cool the mixture. Stuff this mixture into the gourds. Tie each gourd with a thread so the stuffing does not fall out while cooking.

- Heat the oil for deep frying in a pan. Add the stuffed gourds. Fry them on a medium heat till they turn brown and crispy, turning them frequently.

- Untie the bitter gourds and discard the threads. Serve hot.

Cabbage Kofta Curry

(Cabbage Dumplings in Sauce)

Serves 4

Ingredients
1 large cabbage, grated

250g/9oz besan*

Salt to taste

Refined vegetable oil for deep frying

2 tbsp coriander leaves, to garnish

For the sauce:
3 tbsp refined vegetable oil

3 bay leaves

1 black cardamom

1cm/½in cinnamon

1 clove

1 large onion,

finely chopped

2.5cm/1in root ginger, julienned

3 tomatoes, finely chopped

1 tsp ground coriander

1 tsp ground cumin

Salt to taste

250ml/8fl oz water

Method

- Knead together the cabbage, besan and salt to a soft dough. Divide the dough into walnut-sized balls.
- Heat the oil in a frying pan. Add the balls. Deep fry them on a medium heat till they turn golden brown. Drain and set aside.
- For the sauce, heat the oil in a saucepan. Add the bay leaves, cardamom, cinnamon and clove. Let them splutter for 30 seconds.
- Add the onion and ginger. Fry this mixture on a medium heat till the onion turns translucent.
- Add the tomatoes, ground coriander and ground cumin. Mix well. Fry for 2-3 minutes.
- Add the salt and water. Stir for a minute. Cover with a lid and simmer for 5 minutes.
- Uncover the pan and add the kofta balls. Simmer for 5 more minutes, stirring occasionally.
- Garnish with the coriander leaves. Serve hot.

Pineapple Gojju

(Spicy Pineapple Compote)

Serves 4

Ingredients

3 tbsp refined vegetable oil

250ml/8fl oz water

1 tsp mustard seeds

6 curry leaves, crushed

Pinch of asafoetida

½ tsp turmeric

Salt to taste

400g/14oz pineapple, chopped

For the spice mixture:

4 tbsp fresh coconut, grated

3 green chillies

2 red chillies

½ tsp fennel seeds

½ tsp fenugreek seeds

1 tsp cumin seeds

2 tsp coriander seeds

1 small bunch coriander leaves

1 clove

2-3 peppercorns

Method

- Mix all the spice mixture ingredients together.
- Heat 1 tbsp of the oil in a saucepan. Add the spice mixture. Fry it on a medium heat for 1-2 minutes, stirring frequently. Remove from the heat and grind with half the water to a smooth paste. Set aside.
- Heat the remaining oil in a saucepan. Add the mustard seeds and curry leaves. Let them splutter for 15 seconds.
- Add the asafoetida, turmeric and salt. Fry for a minute.
- Add the pineapple, the spice mixture paste and the remaining water. Mix well. Cover with a lid and simmer for 8-12 minutes. Serve hot.

Bitter Gourd Gojju

(Spicy Bitter Gourd Compote)

Serves 4

Ingredients

Salt to taste

4 large bitter gourds*, peeled, slit lengthways, deseeded and sliced

6 tbsp refined vegetable oil

1 tsp mustard seeds

8-10 curry leaves

1 large onion, grated

3-4 garlic cloves, crushed

2 tsp chilli powder

1 tsp ground cumin

½ tsp turmeric

1 tsp ground coriander

2 tsp sambhar powder*

2 tsp fresh coconut, shredded

1 tsp fenugreek seeds, dry roasted and ground

2 tsp white sesame seeds, dry roasted and ground

2 tbsp jaggery*, melted

½ tsp tamarind paste

250ml/8fl oz water

Pinch of asafoetida

Method

- Rub the salt on the bitter gourd slices. Place them in a bowl and seal it with foil. Set aside for 30 minutes. Squeeze out any excess moisture.
- Heat half the oil in a saucepan. Add the bitter gourds. Fry them on a medium heat till they turn golden brown. Set aside.
- Heat the remaining oil in another saucepan. Add the mustard seeds and curry leaves. Let them splutter for 15 seconds.
- Add the onion and garlic. Fry this mixture on a medium heat till the onion turns brown.
- Add the chilli powder, ground cumin, turmeric, ground coriander, sambhar powder and coconut. Fry for 2-3 minutes.
- Add the remaining ingredients, except the water and asafoetida. Fry for another minute.
- Add the fried bitter gourds, some salt and the water. Mix well. Cover with a lid and simmer for 12-15 minutes.
- Add the asafoetida. Mix well. Serve hot.

Baingan Mirchi ka Salan

(Aubergine and Chilli)

Serves 4

Ingredients

6 whole green peppers

4 tbsp refined vegetable oil

600g/1lb 5oz small aubergines, quartered

4 green chillies

1 tsp sesame seeds

10 cashew nuts

20-25 peanuts

5 black peppercorns

¼ tsp fenugreek seeds

¼ tsp mustard seeds

1 tsp ginger paste

1 tsp garlic paste

1 tsp ground coriander

1 tsp ground cumin

½ tsp turmeric

125g/4½oz yoghurt

2 tsp tamarind paste

3 whole red chillies

Salt to taste

1 litre/1¾ pints water

Method

- Deseed and chop the green peppers into long strips.
- Heat 1 tbsp oil in a saucepan. Add the green peppers and sauté them on a medium heat for 1-2 minutes. Set aside.
- Heat 2 tbsp oil in another saucepan. Add the aubergines and green chillies. Sauté on a medium heat for 2-3 minutes. Set aside.
- Heat a frying pan and dry roast the sesame seeds, cashew nuts, peanuts and peppercorns on a medium heat for 1-2 minutes. Remove from the heat and grind the mixture coarsely.
- Heat the remaining oil in a saucepan. Add the fenugreek seeds, mustard seeds, ginger paste, garlic paste, ground coriander, ground cumin, turmeric and the sesame seeds-cashew nuts mixture. Fry on a medium heat for 2-3 minutes.
- Add the sautéed green peppers, the sautéed aubergines and all the remaining ingredients. Simmer for 10-12 minutes.
- Serve hot.

Chicken with Greens

Ingredients

750g/1lb 10oz chicken, chopped into 8 pieces

50g/1¾oz spinach, finely chopped

25g/scant 1oz fresh fenugreek leaves, finely chopped

100g/3½oz coriander leaves, finely chopped

50g/1¾oz mint leaves, finely chopped

6 green chillies, finely chopped

120ml/4fl oz refined vegetable oil

2-3 large onions, finely sliced

Salt to taste

Method

- Mix all the marinade ingredients together. Marinate the chicken with this mixture for an hour.
- Grind together the spinach, fenugreek leaves, coriander leaves and mint leaves with the green chillies to a smooth paste. Mix this paste with the marinated chicken. Set aside.
- Heat the oil in a saucepan. Add the onions. Fry them on a medium heat till they turn brown.

- Add the chicken mixture and the salt. Mix well. Cover with a lid and cook on a low heat for 40 minutes, stirring occasionally. Serve hot.

For the marinade:

1 tsp garam masala

1 tsp ground coriander

1 tsp ground cumin

200g/7oz yoghurt

¼ tsp turmeric

1 tsp chilli powder

1 tsp ginger paste

1 tsp garlic paste

Chicken Tikka Masala

Serves 4

Ingredients

200g/7oz yoghurt

½ tbsp ginger paste

½ tbsp garlic paste

Dash of orange food colour

2 tbsp refined vegetable oil

500g/1lb 2oz boneless chicken, chopped into bite-sized pieces

1 tbsp butter

6 tomatoes, finely chopped

2 large onions

½ tsp ginger paste

½ tsp garlic paste

½ tsp turmeric

1 tbsp garam masala

1 tsp chilli powder

Salt to taste

1 tbsp coriander leaves, finely chopped

Method

- For the tikka, mix together the yoghurt, ginger paste, garlic paste, food colour and 1 tbsp oil. Marinate the chicken with this mixture for 5 hours.
- Grill the marinated chicken for 10 minutes. Set aside.
- Heat the butter in a saucepan. Add the tomatoes. Fry them on a medium heat for 3-4 minutes. Remove from the heat and blend to a smooth paste. Set aside.
- Grind the onion into a smooth paste.
- Heat the remaining oil in a saucepan. Add the onion paste. Fry it on a medium heat till it turns brown.

- Add the ginger paste and garlic paste. Fry for a minute.
- Add the turmeric, garam masala, chilli powder and the tomato paste. Mix well. Stirfry the mixture for 3-4 minutes.
- Add the salt and the grilled chicken. Mix gently till the sauce coats the chicken.
- Garnish with the coriander leaves. Serve hot.

Spicy Stuffed Chicken in Rich Sauce

Serves 4

Ingredients

½ tsp chilli powder

½ tsp garam masala

4 tsp ginger paste

4 tsp garlic paste

Salt to taste

8 chicken breasts, flattened

4 large onions, finely chopped

5cm/1in root ginger, finely chopped

5 green chillies, finely chopped

200g/7oz khoya*

2 tbsp lemon juice

50g/1¾oz coriander leaves, finely chopped

15 cashew nuts

5 tsp desiccated coconut

30g/1oz flaked almonds

1 tsp saffron, soaked in 1 tbsp milk

150g/5½oz ghee

200g/7oz yoghurt, whisked

Method

- Mix the chilli powder, garam masala, half the ginger paste, half the garlic paste and some salt. Marinate the chicken breasts with this mixture for 2 hours.

- Mix together half the onions with the chopped ginger, green chillies, khoya, lemon juice, salt and half the coriander leaves. Divide this mixture into 8 equal portions.

- Place each portion at the narrower end of each chicken breast and roll inwards to seal the breast. Set aside.

- Preheat the oven to 200°C (400°F, Gas Mark 6). Place the stuffed chicken breasts in a greased tray and roast them for 15-20 minutes till they turn golden brown. Set aside.

- Grind together the cashew nuts and coconut to a smooth paste. Set aside.

- Soak the almonds in the saffron milk mixture. Set aside.

- Heat the ghee in a saucepan. Add the remaining onions. Fry them on a medium heat till they turn translucent. Add the remaining ginger paste and garlic paste. Fry the mixture for a minute.

- Add the cashew nuts-coconut paste. Fry for a minute. Add the yoghurt and the roasted chicken breasts. Mix well. Cook on a low heat for 5-6 minutes, stirring frequently. Add the almond-saffron mixture. Mix gently. Simmer for 5 minutes.

- Garnish with the coriander leaves. Serve hot.

Spicy Chicken Masala

Serves 4

Ingredients

6 whole dry red chillies

2 tbsp coriander seeds

6 green cardamom pods

6 cloves

5cm/2in cinnamon

2 tsp fennel seeds

½ tsp black peppercorns

120ml/4fl oz refined vegetable oil

2 large onions, sliced

1cm/½in root ginger, grated

8 garlic cloves, crushed

2 large tomatoes, finely chopped

3-4 bay leaves

1kg/2¼lb chicken, chopped into 12 pieces

½ tsp turmeric

Salt to taste

500ml/16fl oz water

100g/3½oz coriander leaves, finely chopped

Method

- Mix the red chillies, coriander seeds, cardamom, cloves, cinnamon, fennel seeds and peppercorns together.
- Dry roast the mixture and grind to a powder. Set aside.
- Heat the oil in a saucepan. Add the onions. Fry them on a medium heat till they turn brown.
- Add the ginger and garlic. Fry for a minute.
- Add the tomatoes, bay leaves and the ground red chillies-coriander seeds powder. Continue to fry for 2-3 minutes.
- Add the chicken, turmeric, salt and water. Mix well. Cover with a lid and simmer for 40 minutes, stirring at regular intervals.
- Garnish the chicken with the coriander leaves. Serve hot.

Kashmiri Chicken

Serves 4

Ingredients

2 tbsp malt vinegar

2 tsp chilli flakes

2 tsp mustard seeds

2 tsp cumin seeds

½ tsp black peppercorns

7.5cm/3in cinnamon

10 cloves

75g/2½oz ghee

1kg/2¼lb chicken, chopped into 12 pieces

1 tbsp refined vegetable oil

4 bay leaves

4 medium-sized onions, finely chopped

1 tbsp ginger paste

1 tbsp garlic paste

3 tomatoes, finely chopped

1 tsp turmeric

500ml/16fl oz water

Salt to taste

20 cashew nuts, ground

6 strands saffron soaked in the juice of 1 lemon

Method

- Mix the malt vinegar with the chilli flakes, mustard seeds, cumin seeds, peppercorns, cinnamon and cloves. Grind this mixture to a smooth paste. Set aside.
- Heat the ghee in a saucepan. Add the chicken pieces and fry them on a medium heat till they turn golden brown. Drain and set aside.
- Heat the oil in a saucepan. Add the bay leaves and onions. Fry this mixture on a medium heat till the onions turn brown.
- Add the vinegar paste. Mix well and cook this on a low heat for 7-8 minutes.
- Add the ginger paste and garlic paste. Fry this mixture for a minute.
- Add the tomatoes and turmeric. Mix thoroughly and cook on a medium heat for 2-3 minutes.
- Add the fried chicken, water and salt. Mix well to coat the chicken. Cover with a lid and simmer for 30 minutes, stirring occasionally.
- Add the cashew nuts and saffron. Continue to simmer for 5 minutes. Serve hot.

Rum 'n' Chicken

Ingredients

1 tsp garam masala

1 tsp chilli powder

1kg/2¼lb chicken, chopped into 8 pieces

6 garlic cloves

4 black peppercorns

4 cloves

½ tsp cumin seeds

2.5cm/1in cinnamon

50g/1¾oz fresh coconut, grated

4 almonds

1 green cardamom pod

1 tbsp coriander seeds

300ml/10fl oz water

75g/2½oz ghee

3 large onions, finely chopped

Salt to taste

½ tsp saffron

120ml/4fl oz dark rum

1 tbsp coriander leaves, finely chopped

Method

- Mix together the garam masala and the chilli powder. Marinate the chicken with this mixture for 2 hours.
- Dry roast the garlic, peppercorns, cloves, cumin seeds, cinnamon, coconut, almonds, cardamom and coriander seeds.
- Grind with 60ml/2fl oz water to a smooth paste. Set aside.
- Heat the ghee in a saucepan. Add the onions and fry them on a medium heat till they turn translucent.
- Add the garlic-peppercorn paste. Mix well. Fry the mixture for 3-4 minutes.
- Add the marinated chicken and the salt. Mix well. Continue to fry for 3-4 minutes, stirring occasionally.
- Add 240ml/8fl oz water. Stir gently. Cover with a lid and cook on a low heat for 40 minutes, stirring at regular intervals.
- Add the saffron and rum. Mix well and continue to simmer for 10 minutes.
- Garnish with the coriander leaves. Serve hot.

Chicken Shahjahani

(Chicken in Spicy Gravy)

Serves 4

Ingredients

5 tbsp refined vegetable oil

2 bay leaves

5cm/2in cinnamon

6 green cardamom pods

½ tsp cumin seeds

8 cloves

3 large onions, finely chopped

1 tsp turmeric

1 tsp chilli powder

1 tsp ginger paste

1 tsp garlic paste

Salt to taste

75g/2½oz cashew nuts, ground

150g/5½oz yoghurt, whisked

1kg/2¼lb chicken, chopped into 8 pieces

2 tbsp single cream

¼ tsp ground black cardamom

10g/¼oz coriander leaves, finely chopped

Method

- Heat the oil in a saucepan. Add the bay leaves, cinnamon, cardamom, cumin seeds and cloves. Let them splutter for 15 seconds.
- Add the onions, turmeric and chilli powder. Sauté the mixture on a medium heat for 1-2 minutes.
- Add the ginger paste and garlic paste. Fry for 2-3 minutes, stirring constantly.
- Add the salt and ground cashew nuts. Mix well and fry for another minute.
- Add the yoghurt and the chicken. Stir gently till the mixture coats the chicken pieces.
- Cover with a lid and cook the mixture on a low heat for 40 minutes, stirring at frequent intervals.
- Uncover the pan and add the cream and ground cardamom. Stir gently for 5 minutes.
- Garnish the chicken with the coriander leaves. Serve hot.

Easter Chicken

Serves 4

Ingredients

1 tsp lemon juice

1 tsp ginger paste

1 tsp garlic paste

Salt to taste

1kg/2¼lb chicken, chopped into 8 pieces

2 tbsp coriander seeds

12 garlic cloves

2.5cm/1in root ginger

1 tsp cumin seeds

8 red chillies

4 cloves

2.5cm/1in cinnamon

1 tsp turmeric

1 litre/1¾ pints water

4 tbsp refined vegetable oil

3 large onions, finely chopped

4 green chillies, slit lengthways

3 tomatoes, finely chopped

1 tsp tamarind paste

2 large potatoes, quartered

Method

- Mix the lemon juice, ginger paste, garlic paste and salt together. Marinate the chicken pieces with this mixture for 2 hours.
- Mix the coriander seeds, garlic, ginger, cumin seeds, red chillies, cloves, cinnamon and turmeric together.
- Grind this mixture with half the water to a smooth paste. Set aside.
- Heat the oil in a saucepan. Add the onions. Fry them on a medium heat till they turn translucent.
- Add the green chillies and the coriander seeds-garlic paste. Fry this mixture for 3-4 minutes.
- Add the tomatoes and the tamarind paste. Continue to fry for 2-3 minutes.
- Add the marinated chicken, potatoes and the remaining water. Mix thoroughly. Cover with a lid and simmer for 40 minutes, stirring at regular intervals.
- Serve hot.

Spicy Duck with Potatoes

Ingredients

1 tsp ground coriander

2 tsp chilli powder

¼ tsp turmeric

5cm/2in cinnamon

6 cloves

4 green cardamom pods

1 tsp fennel seeds

60ml/2fl oz refined vegetable oil

4 large onions, thinly sliced

5cm/2in root ginger, shredded

8 garlic cloves

6 green chillies, slit lengthways

3 large potatoes, quartered

1kg/2¼lb duck, chopped into 8-10 pieces

2 tsp malt vinegar

750ml/1¼ pints coconut milk

Salt to taste

1 tsp ghee

1 tsp mustard seeds

2 shallots, sliced

8 curry leaves

Method

- Mix the coriander, chilli powder, turmeric, cinnamon, cloves, cardamom and fennel seeds together. Grind this mixture to a powder. Set aside.
- Heat the oil in a saucepan. Add the onions, ginger, garlic and green chillies. Fry on a medium heat for 2-3 minutes.
- Add the spice mixture powder. Sauté for 2 minutes.
- Add the potatoes. Continue to fry for 3-4 minutes.
- Add the duck, malt vinegar, coconut milk and salt. Stir for 5 minutes. Cover with a lid and cook the mixture on a low heat for 40 minutes, stirring at frequent intervals. Once the duck is cooked, remove from the heat and set aside.
- Heat the ghee in a small saucepan. Add the mustard seeds, shallots and curry leaves. Stir-fry on a high heat for 30 seconds.
- Pour this over the duck. Mix well. Serve hot.

Duck Moile

(Simple Duck Curry)

Serves 4

Ingredients

1kg/2¼lb duck, chopped into 12 pieces

Salt to taste

1 tbsp ground coriander

1 tsp ground cumin

6 black peppercorns

4 cloves

2 green cardamom pods

2.5cm/1in cinnamon

120ml/4fl oz refined vegetable oil

3 large onions, finely chopped

5cm/2in root ginger, finely sliced

3 green chillies, finely chopped

½ tsp sugar

2 tbsp malt vinegar

360ml/12fl oz water

Method

- Marinate the duck pieces with the salt for an hour.

- Mix the ground coriander, ground cumin, peppercorns, cloves, cardamom and cinnamon together. Dry roast this mixture in a frying pan on a medium heat for 1-2 minutes.

- Remove from the heat and grind to a fine powder. Set aside.

- Heat the oil in a saucepan. Add the marinated duck pieces. Fry them on a medium heat till they turn brown. Turn occasionally to make sure that they do not burn. Drain and set aside.

- Heat the same oil and add the onions. Fry them on a medium heat till they turn brown.

- Add the ginger and green chillies. Continue to fry for 1-2 minutes.

- Add the sugar, malt vinegar and the coriander-cumin powder. Stir for 2-3 minutes.

- Add the fried duck pieces along with the water. Mix well. Cover with a lid and simmer for 40 minutes, stirring occasionally.

- Serve hot.

Bharwa Murgh Kaju

(Chicken Stuffed with Cashew Nuts)

Serves 4

Ingredients

3 tsp ginger paste

3 tsp garlic paste

10 cashew nuts, ground

1 tsp chilli powder

1 tsp garam masala

Salt to taste

8 chicken breasts, flattened

4 large onions, finely chopped

200g/7oz khoya*

6 green chillies, finely chopped

25g/scant 1oz mint leaves, finely chopped

25g/scant 1oz coriander leaves, finely chopped

2 tbsp lemon juice

75g/2½oz ghee

75g/2½oz cashew nuts, ground

400g/14oz yoghurt, whisked

2 tsp garam masala

2 tsp saffron, soaked in 2 tbsp warm milk

Salt to taste

Method

- Mix together half the ginger paste and half the garlic paste with the ground cashew nuts, chilli powder, garam masala and some salt.
- Marinate the chicken breasts with this mixture for 30 minutes.
- Mix half the onions with the khoya, green chillies, mint leaves, coriander leaves and lemon juice. Divide this mixture into 8 equal portions.
- Spread out a marinated chicken breast. Place a portion of the onion-khoya mixture on it. Roll like a wrap.

- Repeat this for the rest of the chicken breasts.
- Grease a baking dish and place the stuffed chicken breasts inside, with the loose ends face-down.
- Roast the chicken in an oven at 200°C (400°F, Gas Mark 6) for 20 minutes. Set aside.
- Heat the ghee in a saucepan. Add the remaining onions. Fry them on a medium heat till they turn translucent.

- Add the remaining ginger paste and garlic paste. Fry the mixture for 1-2 minutes.
- Add the ground cashew nuts, yoghurt and garam masala. Stir for 1-2 minutes.
- Add the roasted chicken rolls, saffron mixture and some salt. Mix well. Cover with a lid and cook on a low heat for 15-20 minutes. Serve hot.

Yoghurt Chicken Masala

Serves 4

Ingredients

1kg/2¼lb chicken, chopped into 12 pieces

7.5cm/3in root ginger, grated

10 garlic cloves, crushed

½ tsp chilli powder

½ tsp garam masala

½ tsp turmeric

2 green chillies

Salt to taste

200g/7oz yoghurt

½ tsp cumin seeds

1 tsp coriander seeds

4 cloves

4 black peppercorns

2.5cm/1in cinnamon

4 green cardamom pods

6-8 almonds

5 tbsp ghee

4 medium-sized onions, finely chopped

250ml/8fl oz water

1 tbsp coriander leaves, finely chopped

Method

- Pierce the chicken pieces with a fork. Set aside.
- Mix half the ginger and garlic with the chilli powder, garam masala, turmeric, green chillies and salt. Grind this mixture to a smooth paste. Whisk the paste with the yoghurt.
- Marinate the chicken with this mixture for 4-5 hours. Set aside.
- Heat a saucepan. Dry roast the cumin seeds, coriander seeds, cloves, peppercorns, cinnamon, cardamom and almonds. Set aside.

- Heat 4 tbsp of the ghee in a heavy saucepan. Add the onions. Fry them on a medium heat till they turn translucent.
- Add the remaining ginger and garlic. Fry for 1-2 minutes.
- Remove from the heat and grind this mixture with the dry roasted cumin-coriander mixture to a smooth paste.

- Heat the remaining ghee in a saucepan. Add the paste and fry it on a medium heat for 2-3 minutes.
- Add the marinated chicken and fry for another 3-4 minutes.
- Add the water. Stir gently for a minute. Cover with a lid and simmer for 30 minutes, stirring at regular intervals.
- Garnish with the coriander leaves and serve hot.

Chicken Dhansak

(Chicken cooked the Parsi Way)

Serves 4

Ingredients

75g/2½oz toor dhal*

75g/2½oz mung dhal*

75g/2½oz masoor dhal*

75g/2½oz chana dhal*

1 small aubergine, finely chopped

25g/scant 1oz pumpkin, finely chopped

Salt to taste

1 litre/1¾ pints water

8 black peppercorns

6 cloves

2.5cm/1in cinnamon

Pinch of mace

2 bay leaves

1 star anise

3 dry red chillies

2 tbsp refined vegetable oil

50g/1¾oz coriander leaves, finely chopped

50g/1¾oz fresh fenugreek leaves, finely chopped

50g/1¾oz mint leaves, finely chopped

750g/1lb 10oz boneless chicken, chopped into 12 pieces

1 tsp turmeric

¼ tsp grated nutmeg

1 tbsp garlic paste

1 tbsp ginger paste

1 tbsp tamarind paste

Method

- Mix the dhals with the aubergine, pumpkin, salt and half the water. Cook this mixture in a saucepan on a medium heat for 45 minutes.
- Remove from the heat and blend this mixture to a smooth paste. Set aside.
- Mix the peppercorns, cloves, cinnamon, mace, bay leaves, star anise and red chillies together. Dry roast the mixture on a medium heat for 2-3 minutes. Remove from the heat and grind to a fine powder. Set aside.
- Heat the oil in a saucepan. Add the coriander, fenugreek and mint leaves. Fry them on a medium heat for 1-2 minutes. Remove from the heat and grind to a paste. Set aside.
- Mix the chicken with the turmeric, nutmeg, garlic paste, ginger paste, the dhal paste and the remaining water.

Cook this mixture in a saucepan on a medium heat for 30 minutes, stirring occasionally.

- Add the coriander-fenugreek-mint leaves paste. Cook for 2-3 minutes.
- Add the peppercorn-clove powder and the tamarind paste. Mix well. Stir the mixture on a low heat for 8-10 minutes.
- Serve hot.

Chatpata Chicken

(Tangy Chicken)

Serves 4

Ingredients

500g/1lb 2oz boneless chicken, chopped into small pieces

2 tbsp refined vegetable oil

150g/5½oz cauliflower florets

200g/7oz mushrooms, sliced

1 large carrot, sliced

1 large green pepper, deseeded and chopped

Salt to taste

½ tsp ground black pepper

10-15 curry leaves

5 green chillies, finely chopped

5cm/2in root ginger, finely chopped

10 garlic cloves, finely chopped

4 tbsp tomato purée

4 tbsp coriander leaves, finely chopped

For the marinade:

125g/4½oz yoghurt

1½ tbsp ginger paste

1½ tbsp garlic paste

1 tsp chilli powder

1 tsp garam masala

Salt to taste

Method

- Mix all the marinade ingredients together.
- Marinate the chicken with this mixture for 1 hour.
- Heat half a tbsp of the oil in a saucepan. Add the cauliflower, mushrooms, carrot, green pepper, salt and ground black pepper. Mix well. Fry the mixture on a medium heat for 3-4 minutes. Set aside.
- Heat the remaining oil in another saucepan. Add the curry leaves and green chillies. Fry them on a medium heat for a minute.
- Add the ginger and garlic. Fry for another minute.
- Add the marinated chicken and the fried vegetables. Fry for 4-5 minutes.
- Add the tomato purée. Mix well. Cover with a lid and cook the mixture on a low heat for 40 minutes, stirring occasionally.
- Garnish with the coriander leaves. Serve hot.

Masala Duck in Coconut Milk

Serves 4

Ingredients

1kg/2¼lb duck, chopped into 12 pieces

Refined vegetable oil for deep frying

3 large potatoes, chopped

750ml/1¼ pints water

4 tsp coconut oil

1 large onion, finely sliced

100g/3½oz coconut milk

For the spice mixture:

2 tsp ground coriander

½ tsp turmeric

1 tsp ground black pepper

¼ tsp cumin seeds

¼ tsp black cumin seeds

2.5cm/1in cinnamon

9 cloves

2 green cardamom pods

8 garlic cloves

2.5cm/1in root ginger

1 tsp malt vinegar

Salt to taste

Method

- Mix the ingredients of the spice mixture together and grind to a smooth paste.
- Marinate the duck with this paste for 2-3 hours.
- Heat the oil in a saucepan. Add the potatoes and fry them on a medium heat till they turn golden brown. Drain and set aside.
- Heat the water in a saucepan. Add the marinated duck pieces and simmer for 40 minutes, stirring occasionally. Set aside.
- Heat the coconut oil in a frying pan. Add the onion and fry on a medium heat till brown.
- Add the coconut milk. Cook the mixture for 2 minutes, stirring frequently.
- Remove from the heat and add this mixture to the boiled duck. Mix well and simmer for 5-10 minutes.
- Garnish with the fried potatoes. Serve hot.

Chicken Dil Bahar

(Creamy Chicken)

Serves 4

Ingredients

4-5 tbsp refined vegetable oil

2 bay leaves

5cm/2in cinnamon

3 green cardamom pods

4 cloves

2 large onions, finely chopped

1 tsp ginger paste

1 tsp garlic paste

2 tsp ground cumin

2 tsp ground coriander

½ tsp turmeric

4 green chillies, slit lengthways

750g/1lb 10oz boneless chicken, chopped into 16 pieces

50g/1¾oz spring onions, finely chopped

1 large green pepper, finely chopped

1 tsp garam masala

Salt to taste

150g/5½oz tomato purée

125g/4½oz yoghurt

250ml/8fl oz water

2 tbsp butter

85g/3oz cashew nuts

500ml/16fl oz condensed milk

250ml/8fl oz single cream

1 tbsp coriander leaves, finely chopped

Method

- Heat the oil in a saucepan. Add the bay leaves, cinnamon, cardamom and cloves. Let them splutter for 30 seconds.
- Add the onions, ginger paste and garlic paste. Fry this mixture on a medium heat till the onions are brown.
- Add the ground cumin, ground coriander, turmeric and green chillies. Fry the mixture for 2-3 minutes.
- Add the chicken pieces. Mix well. Fry them for 5 minutes.
- Add the spring onions, green pepper, garam masala and salt. Continue to fry for 3-4 minutes.
- Add the tomato purée, yoghurt and water. Mix well and cover with a lid. Cook the mixture on a low heat for 30 minutes, stirring occasionally.

- While the chicken mixture is cooking, heat the butter in another saucepan. Add the cashew nuts and fry them on a medium heat till they turn golden brown. Set aside.

- Add the condensed milk and cream to the chicken mixture. Mix well and continue to simmer for 5 minutes.

- Add the butter with the fried cashew nuts and mix thoroughly for 2 minutes.

- Garnish with the coriander leaves. Serve hot.

Dum ka Murgh

(Slow-cooked Chicken)

Serves 4

Ingredients

4 tbsp refined vegetable oil plus extra for deep frying

3 large onions, sliced

10 almonds

10 cashew nuts

1 tbsp desiccated coconut

1 tsp ginger paste

1 tsp garlic paste

½ tsp turmeric

1 tsp chilli powder

Salt to taste

200g/7oz yoghurt

1kg/2¼lb chicken, finely chopped

1 tbsp coriander leaves, roughly chopped

1 tbsp mint leaves, roughly chopped

½ tsp saffron

Method

- Heat the oil for deep frying. Add the onions and deep fry them on a medium heat till they turn golden brown. Drain and set aside.

- Mix together the almonds, cashew nuts and coconut. Dry roast the mixture. Grind with enough water to form a smooth paste.

- Heat 4 tbsp of the oil in a saucepan. Add the ginger paste, garlic paste, turmeric and chilli powder. Fry on a medium heat for 1-2 minutes.

- Add the almonds-cashew nut paste, the fried onions, the salt and yoghurt. Cook for 4-5 minutes.

- Transfer to an ovenproof dish. Add the chicken, coriander and mint leaves. Mix thoroughly.

- Sprinkle the saffron on top. Seal with foil and cover tightly with a lid. Bake in an oven at 180°C (350°F, Gas Mark 4) for 40 minutes.

- Serve hot.

Murgh Kheema Masala

(Spicy Minced Chicken)

Serves 4

Ingredients

60ml/2fl oz refined vegetable oil

5cm/2in cinnamon

4 cloves

2 green cardamom pods

½ tsp cumin seeds

2 large onions, finely chopped

1 tsp ground coriander

½ tsp ground cumin

½ tsp turmeric

1 tsp chilli powder

2 tsp ginger paste

3 tsp garlic paste

3 tomatoes, finely chopped

200g/7oz frozen peas

1kg/2¼lb chicken mince

75g/2½oz cashew nuts, ground

125g/4½oz yoghurt

250ml/8fl oz water

Salt to taste

4 tbsp single cream

25g/scant 1oz coriander leaves, finely chopped

Method

- Heat the oil in a saucepan. Add the cinnamon, cloves, cardamom and cumin seeds. Let them splutter for 15 seconds.
- Add the onions, ground coriander, ground cumin, turmeric and chilli powder. Fry on a medium heat for 1-2 minutes.
- Add the ginger paste and garlic paste. Continue to fry for a minute.
- Add the tomatoes, peas and chicken mince. Mix well. Cook this mixture on a low heat for 10-15 minutes, stirring occasionally.
- Add the yoghurt, water and salt. Mix well. Cover with a lid and simmer for 20-25 minutes.
- Garnish with the cream and coriander leaves. Serve hot.

Stuffed Chicken Nawabi

Serves 4

Ingredients

200g/7oz yoghurt

2 tbsp lemon juice

½ tsp turmeric

Salt to taste

1kg/2¼lb chicken

100g/3½oz breadcrumbs

For the stuffing:

120ml/4fl oz refined vegetable oil

1½ tsp ginger paste

1½ tsp garlic paste

2 large onions, finely chopped

2 green chillies, finely chopped

½ tsp chilli powder

1 chicken gizzard, chopped

1 chicken liver, chopped

200g/7oz peas

2 carrots, diced

50g/1¾oz coriander leaves, finely chopped

2 tbsp mint leaves, finely chopped

½ tsp ground black pepper

½ tsp garam masala

20 cashew nuts, chopped

20 raisins

Method

- Whisk the yoghurt with the lemon juice, turmeric and salt. Marinate the chicken with this mixture for 1-2 hours.
- For the stuffing, heat the oil in a saucepan. Add the ginger paste, garlic paste and onions and fry them on a medium heat for 1-2 minutes.
- Add the green chillies, chilli powder, chicken gizzard and chicken liver. Mix well. Fry for 3-4 minutes.
- Add the peas, carrots, coriander leaves, mint leaves, pepper, garam masala, cashew nuts and raisins. Stir for 2 minutes. Cover with a lid and cook on a low heat for 20 minutes, stirring occasionally.
- Remove from the heat and set aside to cool.
- Stuff this mixture into the marinated chicken.
- Roll the stuffed chicken in the breadcrumbs and roast in a preheated oven at 200°C (400°F, Gas Mark 6) for 50 minutes.
- Serve hot.

Murgh ke Nazare

(Chicken with Cheddar Cheese and Paneer)

Serves 4

Ingredients

Salt to taste

½ tbsp ginger paste

½ tbsp garlic paste

Juice of 1 lemon

750g/1lb 10oz boneless chicken pieces, flattened

75g/2½oz paneer*, grated

250g/9oz chicken mince

75g/2½oz Cheddar cheese, grated

1 tsp ground coriander

½ tsp garam masala

½ tsp turmeric

125g/4½oz khoya*

1 tsp chilli powder

2 eggs, boiled and finely chopped

3 tomatoes, finely chopped

2 green chillies, finely chopped

2 large onions, finely chopped

2 tbsp coriander leaves, chopped

½ tsp ginger powder

For the sauce:

4 tbsp refined vegetable oil

½ tbsp ginger paste

½ tbsp garlic paste

2 large onions, ground

2 green chillies, finely chopped

½ tsp turmeric

1 tsp ground coriander

½ tsp ground white pepper

½ tsp ground cumin

½ tsp dry ginger powder

200g/7oz yoghurt

4 cashew nuts, ground

4 almonds, ground

125g/4½oz khoya*

Method

- Mix the salt, ginger paste, garlic paste and lemon juice together. Marinate the chicken with this mixture for 1 hour. Set aside.

- Mix the paneer with the chicken mince, cheese, ground coriander, garam masala, turmeric and khoya.

- Spread this mixture over the marinated chicken. Sprinkle the chilli powder, eggs, tomatoes, green chillies, onions, coriander leaves and ginger powder on top of it. Roll the chicken like a wrap and seal by tying it tightly with a string.

- Bake in an oven at 200°C (400°F, Gas Mark 6) for 30 minutes. Set aside.

- For the sauce, heat the oil in a saucepan. Add the ginger paste, garlic paste, onions and green chillies. Fry them on a medium heat for 2-3 minutes. Add the remaining sauce ingredients. Cook for 7-8 minutes.

- Slice the chicken roll into bite-sized pieces and arrange in a serving dish. Pour the sauce over them. Serve hot.

Murgh Pasanda

(Spicy Chicken Bites)

Serves 4

Ingredients

1 tsp turmeric

30g/1oz coriander leaves, chopped

1 tsp chilli powder

10g/¼oz mint leaves, finely chopped

1 tsp garam masala

5cm/2in piece of raw papaya, ground

1 tsp ginger paste

1 tsp garlic paste

Salt to taste

750g/1lb 10oz chicken breast, chopped into thin slices

6 tbsp refined vegetable oil

Method

- Mix all the ingredients, except the chicken and oil. Marinate the chicken slices with this mixture for 3 hours.

- Heat the oil in a frying pan. Add the marinated chicken slices and fry on a medium heat till golden brown, turning occasionally. Serve hot.

Murgh Masala

(Chicken Masala)

Serves 4

Ingredients

4 tbsp refined vegetable oil

2 large onions, grated

1 tomato, finely chopped

Salt to taste

1kg/2¼lb chicken, chopped into 8 pieces

360ml/12fl oz water

360ml/12fl oz coconut milk

For the spice mixture:

2 tbsp garam masala

1 tsp cumin seeds

1½ tsp poppy seeds

4 red chillies

½ tsp turmeric

8 garlic cloves

2.5cm/1in root ginger

Method

- Grind the spice mixture with enough water to form a smooth paste. Set aside.
- Heat the oil in a saucepan. Add the onions and fry on a medium heat till brown. Add the spice mixture paste and fry for 5-6 minutes.
- Add the tomato, salt, chicken and water. Cover with a lid and simmer for 20 minutes. Add the coconut milk, mix well and serve hot.

Bohri Chicken Cream

(Chicken in Creamy Gravy)

Serves 4

Ingredients

3 large onions

2.5cm/1in root ginger

8 garlic cloves

6 green chillies

100g/3½oz coriander leaves, finely chopped

3 tbsp mint leaves, finely chopped

120ml/4fl oz water

1kg/2¼lb chicken, chopped into 8 pieces

2 tbsp lemon juice

1 tsp ground black pepper

250ml/8fl oz single cream

30g/1oz ghee

Salt to taste

Method

- Mix the onions, ginger, garlic, green chillies, coriander leaves and mint leaves together. Grind this mixture with the water to make a fine paste.
- Marinate the chicken with half this paste and the lemon juice for 1 hour.
- Place the marinated chicken in a saucepan and pour the remaining paste over it. Sprinkle the remaining ingredients on top of this mixture.
- Seal with foil, cover tightly with a lid and cook on a low heat for 45 minutes. Serve hot.

Jhatpat Murgh

(Quick Chicken)

Serves 4

Ingredients

4 tbsp refined vegetable oil

2 large onions, finely sliced

2 tsp ginger paste

Salt to taste

1kg/2¼lb chicken, chopped into 12 pieces

¼ tsp saffron, dissolved in 2 tbsp milk

Method

- Heat the oil in a saucepan. Add the onions and ginger paste. Fry them on a medium heat for 2 minutes.
- Add the salt and chicken. Cook on a low heat for 30 minutes, stirring frequently. Sprinkle with the saffron mixture. Serve hot.

Green Chicken Curry

Serves 4

Ingredients

Salt to taste

A pinch of turmeric

Juice of 1 lemon

1kg/2¼lb chicken, chopped into 12 pieces

3.5cm/1½in root ginger

8 garlic cloves

100g/3½oz coriander leaves, chopped

3 green chillies

4 tbsp refined vegetable oil

2 large onions, grated

½ tsp garam masala

250ml/8fl oz water

Method

- Mix the salt, turmeric and lemon juice. Marinate the chicken with this mixture for 30 minutes.

- Grind the ginger, garlic, coriander leaves and chillies to a smooth paste.

- Heat the oil in a saucepan. Add the paste along with the grated onions and fry on a medium heat for 2-3 minutes.

- Add the marinated chicken, garam masala and water. Mix well and simmer for 40 minutes, stirring frequently. Serve hot.

Murgh Bharta

(Stewed Chicken with Eggs)

Serves 4

Ingredients

4 tbsp refined vegetable oil

2 large onions, finely sliced

500g/1lb 2oz boneless chicken, diced

1 tsp garam masala

½ tsp turmeric

Salt to taste

3 tomatoes, finely sliced

30g/1oz coriander leaves, chopped

4 hard-boiled eggs, halved

Method

- Heat the oil in a saucepan. Fry the onions on a medium heat till brown. Add the chicken, garam masala, turmeric and salt. Fry for 5 minutes.
- Add the tomatoes. Mix well and cook on a low heat for 30-40 minutes. Garnish with the coriander leaves and eggs. Serve hot.

Chicken with Ajowan Seeds

Serves 4

Ingredients

3 tbsp refined vegetable oil

1½ tsp ajowan seeds

2 large onions, finely chopped

1 tsp ginger paste

1 tsp garlic paste

4 tomatoes, finely chopped

2 tsp ground coriander

1 tsp chilli powder

1 tsp turmeric

1kg/2¼lb chicken, chopped into 8 pieces

250ml/8fl oz water

Juice of 1 lemon

1 tsp garam masala

Salt to taste

Method

- Heat the oil in a saucepan. Add the ajowan seeds. Let them splutter for 15 seconds.

- Add the onions and fry on a medium heat till brown. Add the ginger paste, garlic paste and tomatoes. Fry for 3 minutes, stirring occasionally.

- Add all the remaining ingredients. Mix well and cover with a lid. Simmer for 40 minutes and serve hot.

Spinach Chicken Tikka

Serves 4

Ingredients

1kg/2¼lb boneless chicken, chopped into 16 pieces

2 tbsp ghee

1 tsp chaat masala*

2 tbsp lemon juice

For the marinade:

100g/3½oz spinach, ground

50g/1¾oz coriander leaves, ground

1 tsp ginger paste

1 tsp garlic paste

200g/7oz yoghurt

1½ tsp garam masala

Method

- Mix all the ingredients for the marinade. Marinate the chicken with this mixture for 2 hours.
- Baste the chicken with the ghee and roast in an oven at 200°C (400°F, Gas Mark 6) for 45 minutes. Sprinkle the chaat masala and lemon juice on top. Serve hot.

Yakhni Chicken

(Kashmiri-style Chicken)

Serves 4

Ingredients

3 tbsp refined vegetable oil

1kg/2¼lb chicken, chopped into 8 pieces

400g/14oz yoghurt

125g/4½oz besan*

2 cloves

2.5cm/1in cinnamon

6 peppercorns

1 tsp ground ginger

2 tsp ground fennel

Salt to taste

250ml/8fl oz water

50g/1¾oz coriander leaves, chopped

Method

- Heat half the oil in a frying pan. Add the chicken pieces and fry them on a medium heat till they turn golden brown. Set aside.

- Whisk the yoghurt with the besan to form a thick paste. Set aside.

- Heat the remaining oil in a saucepan. Add the cloves, cinnamon, peppercorns, ground ginger, ground fennel and salt. Fry for 4-5 minutes.

- Add the fried chicken, water and the yoghurt paste. Mix well and simmer for 40 minutes. Garnish with the coriander leaves. Serve hot.

Chilli Chicken

Serves 4

Ingredients

3 tbsp refined vegetable oil

4 green chillies, finely chopped

1 tsp ginger paste

1 tsp garlic paste

3 large onions, sliced

250ml/8fl oz water

750g/1lb 10oz boneless chicken, chopped

2 large green peppers, julienned

2 tbsp soy sauce

30g/1oz coriander leaves, chopped

Salt to taste

Method

- Heat the oil in a saucepan. Add the green chillies, ginger paste, garlic paste and onions. Fry on a medium heat for 3-4 minutes.
- Add the water and chicken. Simmer for 20 minutes.
- Add all the remaining ingredients and cook for 20 minutes. Serve hot.

Pepper Chicken

Serves 4

Ingredients

4 tbsp refined vegetable oil

3 large onions, finely chopped

6 garlic cloves, finely chopped

1kg/2¼lb chicken, chopped into 12 pieces

3 tsp ground coriander

2½ tsp freshly ground black pepper

½ tsp turmeric

Salt to taste

250ml/8fl oz water

Juice of 1 lemon

50g/1¾oz coriander leaves, chopped

Method

- Heat the oil in a saucepan. Add the onions and garlic and fry on a medium heat till brown.
- Add the chicken. Fry for 5 minutes, stirring frequently.
- Add the ground coriander, pepper, turmeric and salt. Fry for 3-4 minutes.

- Pour in the water, mix well and cover with a lid. Simmer for 40 minutes.
- Garnish with the lemon juice and coriander leaves. Serve hot.

Chicken with Figs

Serves 4

Ingredients

4 tbsp refined vegetable oil

2 large onions, finely chopped

1 tsp ginger paste

1 tsp garlic paste

1kg/2¼lb chicken, chopped into 12 pieces

250ml/8fl oz warm water

200g/7oz tomato purée

Salt to taste

2 tsp malt vinegar

12 dry figs, soaked for 2 hours

Method

- Heat the oil in a frying pan. Add the onions. Fry them on a medium heat till translucent. Add the ginger paste and garlic paste. Fry for 2-3 minutes.
- Add the chicken and water. Cover with a lid and simmer for 30 minutes.
- Add the tomato purée, salt and vinegar. Mix well. Drain the figs and add them to the chicken mixture. Simmer for 8-10 minutes. Serve hot.

Mutton Biryani

Ingredients

1kg/2¼lb mutton, cut into 5cm/2in pieces

360ml/12fl oz refined vegetable oil

2 large potatoes, quartered

4 cloves

5cm/2in cinnamon

3 bay leaves

6 peppercorns

2 black cardamom pods

Salt to taste

3 tbsp ghee

750g/1lb 10oz basmati rice, parboiled

A large pinch of saffron, dissolved in 1 tbsp milk

For the marinade:

100g/3½oz coriander leaves, ground to a paste

50g/1¾oz mint leaves, ground to a paste

200g/7oz beaten yoghurt

1½ tsp ginger paste

1½ tsp garlic paste

3 green chillies, finely chopped

1½ tsp garam masala

1 tsp ground cumin

1 tsp ground coriander

4 large onions, chopped and deep fried

Method

- Mix all the marinade ingredients together and marinate the mutton with this mixture overnight in the refrigerator.
- Heat 250ml/8fl oz oil in a saucepan. Add the potatoes and fry them on a medium heat for 10 minutes. Drain and set aside.
- Heat the remaining oil in a large saucepan. Add the cloves, cinnamon, bay leaves, peppercorns and cardamom. Let them splutter for 30 seconds.
- Add the marinated mutton and salt. Simmer for 45 minutes, stirring occasionally. Add the fried potatoes. Stir lightly. Remove from the heat.
- Pour the ghee in a saucepan. Place the meat-potatoes mixture in the saucepan. Arrange the parboiled rice in a layer over the meat-potatoes mixture.
- Pour the saffron milk on top. Seal with foil and cover with a tight lid. Cook on a low heat for 20 minutes.
- Serve hot.

Faada-ni-Khichdi

(Cracked Wheat Porridge)

Serves 4

Ingredients

125g/4½oz cracked wheat

150g/5½oz mung dhal*

150g/5½oz masoor dhal*

2 litres/3½ pints water

2 tomatoes, puréed

100g/3½oz frozen mixed vegetables

½ tsp turmeric

½ tsp chilli powder

½ tsp ground coriander

½ tsp ground cumin

2 green chillies, finely chopped

Salt to taste

4 tbsp ghee

2 cloves

2.5cm/1in cinnamon

6 black peppercorns

2 bay leaves

8 curry leaves

3 tbsp coriander leaves, finely chopped

1 tsp cumin seeds, dry-roasted and ground

Method

- Mix the cracked wheat, dhals and the water in a saucepan and bring to a boil on a high heat. Cook the mixture on a low heat for 30 minutes.
- Add the tomato purée, mixed vegetables, turmeric, chilli powder, ground coriander, cumin, chillies and salt. Stir well and simmer for 5 minutes.
- Heat the ghee in a small pan. Add the cloves, cinnamon, peppercorns, bay leaves and curry leaves. Let them splutter for 15 seconds.
- Pour this seasoning in the cooked wheat mixture and let it simmer for 3-5 minutes.
- Garnish the khichdi with the coriander leaves and ground cumin. Serve hot.

Urad Dhal Roti

(Split Black Gram Bread)

Makes 15

Ingredients

600g/1lb 5oz urad dhal*, soaked overnight

2 tbsp ghee

1 tsp turmeric

1 tsp ginger powder

1 tsp ground coriander

¼ tsp chilli powder

350g/12oz plain white flour

1 tsp crushed anardana*

2 tbsp coriander leaves, finely chopped

3 green chillies, finely chopped

1 small onion, grated

Salt to taste

120ml/4fl oz water

Method

- Drain the dhal and grind to a thick paste.
- Heat the ghee in a frying pan. Add the dhal paste along with the turmeric, ginger powder, coriander and chilli powder. Fry on a medium heat for 4-5 minutes. Cool for 5 minutes and divide into 15 portions. Set aside.
- Knead all the remaining ingredients to form a stiff dough. Divide into 15 balls and roll out into discs, 10cm/4in in diameter.
- Place a portion of the dhal mixture on each disc, seal and roll out again into discs, 15cm/6in in diameter.
- Grease and heat a flat pan. Cook a roti till the underside is brown. Flip and repeat. Cook each side twice.
- Repeat for the rest of the rotis.
- Serve hot.

Murgh-Methi-Malai Paratha

(Chicken and Fenugreek Pan-fried Bread)

Makes 14

Ingredients

4 tsp refined vegetable oil

½ tsp cumin seeds

6 garlic cloves, finely chopped

1 large onion, finely chopped

4 green chillies, finely chopped

1cm/½in root ginger, finely chopped

½ tsp chilli powder

½ tsp garam masala

200g/7oz chicken, minced

60g/2oz fresh fenugreek leaves, finely chopped

1 tsp lemon juice

1 tbsp coriander leaves, finely chopped

750g/1lb 10oz wholemeal flour

Salt to taste

360ml/12fl oz water

Ghee for greasing

Method

- Heat half the oil in a saucepan. Add the cumin seeds, garlic, onion, green chillies, ginger, chilli powder and garam masala. Let them splutter for 30 seconds.

- Add the chicken, fenugreek, lemon juice and coriander leaves. Mix well. Cook on a medium heat for 30 minutes, stirring occasionally. Set aside.

- Knead the flour, salt and the remaining oil with the water to form a stiff dough. Divide into 14 balls and roll out into discs of 10cm/4in diameter.

- Place a spoonful of the chicken mixture on each disc, seal and roll out carefully into discs of 12.5cm/5in diameter.

- Heat a flat pan and cook a paratha on a low heat till the underside is light brown. Smear some ghee on the top, flip and repeat. Cook each side twice.

- Repeat for the remaining parathas. Serve hot.

Meethi Puri

(Sweet Puffed Bread)

Makes 20

Ingredients

250g/9oz sugar

60ml/2fl oz warm water

350g/12oz plain white flour

2 tbsp ghee

1 tbsp Greek yoghurt

Salt to taste

Refined vegetable oil for deep frying

Method

- Cook the sugar and water in a saucepan on a medium heat till it achieves a 1-thread consistency. Set aside.
- Mix all the remaining ingredients, except the oil, together. Cook in a saucepan on a medium heat for 3-4 minutes. Knead into a stiff dough.
- Divide into 20 balls. Roll out into discs, 7.5cm/3in in diameter.

- Heat the oil. Deep fry the puris on a medium heat till golden brown.
- Drain and toss the fried puris in the sugar syrup. Serve hot.

Kulcha

(Baked Flat Bread)

Makes 8

Ingredients

1 tsp dry yeast, dissolved in 120ml/4fl oz warm water

½ tsp salt

90ml/3fl oz water

350g/12oz plain white flour

1 tsp bicarbonate of soda

60ml/2fl oz warm milk

4 tbsp sour cream

1 tbsp refined vegetable oil

Ghee for greasing

Method

- Mix the yeast with the salt. Set aside for 10 minutes.
- Knead with all the remaining ingredients, except the ghee, to form a firm dough. Cover with a wet cloth. Set aside for 5 hours.
- Divide into 8 balls and roll out into teardrop shapes.
- Grease and heat a flat pan. Cook each kulcha on a low heat for a minute. Flip and repeat. Serve hot.

Garlic & Cheese Naan

(Garlic and Cheese Naan Bread)

Makes 8

Ingredients

15 garlic cloves, finely chopped

85g/3oz Cheddar cheese, grated

350g/12oz plain white flour

¼ tsp baking powder

1 tbsp dry yeast, dissolved in 120ml/4fl oz warm water

2 tbsp plain yoghurt

2 tbsp sugar

Salt to taste

120ml/4fl oz water

Refined vegetable oil for greasing

Method

- Knead all the ingredients together to form a dough.
- Grease and heat a flat pan. Spread a large spoonful of the batter like a thick pancake.
- Cook till the underside is brown. Flip and repeat.
- Repeat for the remaining batter. Serve hot.

Tri-flour Roti

Makes 14

Ingredients

175g/6oz wholemeal flour

175g/6oz soy flour

175g/6oz millet flour

1 tsp ground coriander

½ tsp ground cumin

½ tsp chilli powder

½ tsp turmeric

2 tsp refined vegetable oil

Salt to taste

250ml/8fl oz water

Method

- Knead all the ingredients to form a pliable dough.
- Divide into 14 balls and roll out into discs 15cm/6in in diameter.
- Heat a flat pan and cook each roti on both sides, flipping every 30 seconds, till each side is golden brown.
- Serve hot.

Sheera Chapatti

(Sweet Semolina Flat Bread)

Makes 10

Ingredients

350g/12oz plain white flour

250ml/8fl oz water

3 tbsp ghee

150g/5½oz semolina

250g/9oz jaggery*, grated

1 tbsp ground green cardamom

Method

- Knead the flour with half the water to form a stiff dough. Divide into 10 balls. Set aside.
- Heat half a tbsp of ghee in a saucepan. Fry the semolina on a medium heat till golden brown. Add the remaining water and stir till it evaporates.
- Add the jaggery and cardamom. Mix well and cook for 3-4 minutes.
- Cool the mixture for 10 minutes, then divide into 10 portions.

- Flatten each dough ball and place a portion of semolina in the centre of each. Seal and roll out into discs 12.5cm/5in in diameter.

- Grease and heat a flat pan. Cook a chapatti on a low heat till the underside is golden brown.

- Smear some ghee on the top, flip and repeat. Cook each side twice.

- Repeat for the remaining chapattis. Serve hot.

Bhakri

(Plain Flat Bread)

Makes 8

Ingredients

350g/12oz millet flour

Salt to taste

120ml/4fl oz warm water

1 tbsp ajowan seeds

Method

- Knead all the ingredients to form a soft dough. Divide into 8 balls and pat to flatten into discs 15cm/6in in diameter.
- Heat a flat pan, place a bhakri on the pan and spread a tsp of water over it. Flip and cook till the underside is brown. Cook each side twice.
- Repeat for the remaining bhakri. Serve hot.

Chapatti

(Pan-baked Puffed Bread)

Makes 10

Ingredients

350g/12oz wholemeal flour

½ tsp salt

2 tsp refined vegetable oil

120ml/4fl oz water

Method

- Knead all the ingredients to form a soft, pliable dough.
- Divide into 10 balls. Roll out with a flour-coated rolling pin into thin tortilla-like discs.
- Grease and heat a flat pan. Spread out a chapatti on the pan and cook on a low heat till the underside is light brown. Flip and repeat.
- Repeat for the rest of the chapattis.
- Serve hot.

Rice & Coconut Roti

(Rice and Coconut Bread)

Makes 8

Ingredients

175g/6oz rice flour

25g/scant 1oz coriander leaves, finely chopped

60g/2oz fresh coconut, grated

1 tsp refined vegetable oil

1 tsp cumin seeds

Salt to taste

90ml/3fl oz warm water

Method

- Knead all the ingredients together to form a pliable dough. Divide into 8 balls. Roll out into discs 15cm/6in in diameter.
- Heat a flat pan and cook a roti on a low heat till the underside is brown.
- Smear some oil on top, flip and repeat. Cook each side twice.
- Repeat for the remaining rotis. Serve hot.

Egg Paratha

(Pan-fried Bread with Egg)

Makes 10

Ingredients

350g/12oz wholemeal flour

120ml/4fl oz water

4 eggs, whisked

1 small onion, finely chopped

4 green chillies, finely chopped

10g/¼oz coriander leaves, finely chopped

1 tomato, finely chopped

¾ tsp salt

150ml/5fl oz refined vegetable oil

Method

- Knead the flour with the water to form a firm dough. Divide into 10 balls. Roll out into 10 discs of 15cm/6in diameter.
- Mix the remaining ingredients, except the oil, together. Set aside.

- Heat a flat pan and cook a paratha on a low heat for 2-3 minutes. Flip over and spread 1 tbsp of the egg mixture on the cooked side of the disc. Pour 1 tbsp oil over it.
- Gently flip and cook, egg-side-down, for 30 seconds. Carefully remove from the flat pan with a spatula.
- Repeat for the remaining parathas. Serve hot.